Copyright © 2023 by Monica Dimitrios

Contents

The hormonal changes of menopause might make you more likely to gain weight around your abdomen than around your hips and thighs. But, hormonal changes alone don't necessarily cause menopause weight gain. Instead, the weight gain is usually related to aging, as well as lifestyle and genetic factors.

Menopause brings with it a list of annoying and sometimes unpleasant symptoms but you can make your transition easier by picking the best foods for menopause. We're not saying that improved nutrition is a complete one-size-fits-all solution for menopause, but it's a good place to start if you want to find trigger patterns and alleviate symptoms. On top of this, what you eat at menopause can help reduce the long-term effects of lower oestrogen levels, such as the risk of cardiovascular disease and osteoporosis.

1. Linguine with Creamy Mushroom Sauce

Prep Time: 40 mins

Total Time: 40 mins

Servings: 4

Ingredients

- 8 ounces whole-wheat linguine pasta
- 2 tablespoons extra-virgin olive oil
- 6 cloves garlic, sliced
- 1 ½ pounds mixed mushrooms, sliced
- 1 cup diced shallots
- 1 tablespoon chopped fresh thyme
- 1 cup dry white wine
- ½ cup sour cream or crème fraîche
- ¼ cup grated Parmesan cheese plus more for garnish
- 1 tablespoon butter
- ½ teaspoon salt
- ¼ teaspoon ground pepper
- Finely chopped fresh parsley for garnish

Directions

1. Bring a large pot of water to a boil over high heat. Cook pasta according to package directions. Reserve 1/2 cup of the pasta water, then drain the pasta.

2. Meanwhile, heat oil and garlic in a large skillet over medium heat until fragrant, about 2 minutes. Add mushrooms, shallots and thyme and increase heat to high. Cook, stirring occasionally, until the liquid the mushrooms release has evaporated and the mushrooms are starting to brown, 11 to 13 minutes.

3. Add wine to the pan and cook until it is reduced by about half, about 3 minutes. Stir in the reserved pasta water, sour cream (or crème fraîche), Parmesan, butter, salt and pepper. Add the pasta and toss to coat. Serve topped with more Parmesan and parsley, if desired.

Prep Time: 15 mins

Total Time: 30 mins

Servings: 4

Ingredients

- 12 ounces new potatoes, quartered
- 2 bunches scallions, trimmed
- 4 tablespoons extra-virgin olive oil, divided
- ¾ teaspoon ground pepper, divided
- ½ teaspoon salt, divided
- 4 large boneless, skinless chicken thighs (1-1 1/4 pounds), trimmed
- 2 tablespoons sherry vinegar
- 2 tablespoons chopped fresh herbs, such as dill, thyme and/or parsley
- 1 tablespoon whole-grain mustard
- 1 tablespoon finely chopped shallot

Directions

1. Preheat oven to 450 degrees F.

2. Toss potatoes and scallions with 4 teaspoons oil and 1/4 teaspoon each pepper and salt in a large bowl. Spread evenly on a large rimmed baking sheet. Place chicken on top; drizzle with 2 teaspoons oil and sprinkle with 1/4 teaspoon each pepper and salt. Roast until an instant-read thermometer inserted into the thickest part registers 165 degrees F and the potatoes are tender, 18 to 20 minutes.

3. Meanwhile, whisk the remaining 2 tablespoons oil and 1/4 teaspoon pepper with vinegar, herbs, mustard and shallot in a small bowl. Serve drizzled over the chicken and vegetables.

3. Cream of Turkey & Wild Rice Soup

Prep Time: 35 mins

Total Time: 35 mins

Servings: 4

Ingredients

- 1 tablespoon extra-virgin olive oil
- 2 cups sliced mushrooms, (about 4 ounces)
- ¾ cup chopped celery
- ¾ cup chopped carrots
- ¼ cup chopped shallots
- ¼ cup all-purpose flour
- ¼ teaspoon salt
- ¼ teaspoon freshly ground pepper
- 4 cups reduced-sodium chicken broth
- 1 cup quick-cooking or instant wild rice
- 3 cups shredded cooked chicken, or turkey
- ½ cup reduced-fat sour cream
- 2 tablespoons chopped fresh parsley

Directions

1. Heat oil in a large saucepan over medium heat. Add mushrooms, celery, carrots and shallots; cook, stirring, until softened, about 5 minutes. Add flour, salt and pepper; cook, stirring, for 2 minutes more.
2. Add broth and bring to a boil, scraping up any browned bits. Add rice and reduce heat to a simmer. Cover and cook until the rice is tender, 5 to 7 minutes. Stir in turkey (or chicken), sour cream and parsley; cook until heated through, about 2 minutes more.

Prep Time: 25 mins

Total Time: 25 mins

Servings: 4

Ingredients

- 1 tablespoon olive oil

- 2 (6 ounce) boneless, skinless chicken breasts

- 2 tablespoons all-purpose flour

- 1 ½ cups reduced-fat milk, divided

- 3 cloves garlic, minced

- 2 ½ cups water

- 6 ounces whole-wheat linguine

- 3 ounces Parmesan cheese, grated (about 3/4 cup)

- 1 tablespoon reduced-fat cream cheese

- ½ teaspoon ground pepper

Directions

1. Heat oil in a large Dutch oven over medium-high heat. Add chicken; cook until browned on both sides, 7 to 8 minutes total. Remove from the pot and cut into 1-inch cubes.

2. Whisk together flour and 1/4 cup milk; set aside.

3. Add garlic to the pot; cook, stirring often, for 1
    minute. Add water and the remaining 1 1/4 cups
    milk; cover and bring to a boil. Add pasta; cover
    and cook, stirring occasionally, for 8 minutes. Stir
    in the chicken and the milk-flour mixture;
    continue to cook until the pasta is al dente, about 3
    minutes more.

4. Remove from heat; add Parmesan, cream cheese
    and pepper; stir until the cheese is melted. Serve
    immediately.

Prep Time: 10 mins

Total Time: 40 mins

Servings: 4

Ingredients

- 1 pound baby Yukon Gold potatoes, halved
- 2 tablespoons extra-virgin olive oil, divided
- ¾ teaspoon salt, divided
- ½ teaspoon ground pepper, divided
- 12 ounces asparagus, trimmed
- 2 tablespoons melted butter
- 1 tablespoon lemon juice
- 2 cloves garlic, minced
- 1 ¼ pounds salmon fillet, skinned and cut into 4 portions
- Chopped parsley for garnish

Directions

1. Preheat oven to 400 degrees F. Toss potatoes, 1 tablespoon oil, 1/4 teaspoon salt and 1/8 teaspoon

pepper together in a medium bowl. Spread in an even layer on a large rimmed baking sheet. Roast until starting to soften and brown, about 15 minutes.

2. Meanwhile, toss asparagus with the remaining 1 tablespoon oil, 1/8 teaspoon salt and 1/8 teaspoon pepper in the medium bowl. Combine butter, lemon juice, garlic, 1/4 teaspoon salt and the remaining 1/4 teaspoon pepper in a small bowl.

3. Sprinkle salmon with the remaining 1/8 teaspoon salt. Move the potatoes to one side of the pan. Place the salmon in the center of the pan; drizzle with the butter mixture. Spread the asparagus on the empty side of the pan. Roast until the salmon is just cooked through and the vegetables are tender, 10 to 12 minutes. Garnish with parsley.

6. Skillet Lasagna

Prep Time: 45 mins

Total Time: 45 mins

Servings: 6

Ingredients

- 1 teaspoon extra-virgin olive oil
- 1 pound 94%-lean ground beef
- 1 teaspoon salt-free Italian seasoning
- ½ teaspoon garlic powder
- ½ teaspoon onion powder
- ½ teaspoon ground pepper
- 2 ½ cups water
- 1 (24 ounce) jar lower-sodium marinara sauce
- 10 uncooked lasagna noodles, preferably whole-wheat, broken into 2-inch pieces
- ¼ cup grated Parmesan cheese
- ¼ cup packed chopped fresh basil, plus more for garnish
- ¼ cup packed chopped fresh parsley
- ¾ cup shredded part-skim mozzarella or provolone cheese

- ½ cup part-skim ricotta cheese

Directions

1. Preheat oven to broil with a rack about 8 inches from the heat source.

2. Heat oil in a large cast-iron or ovenproof skillet over medium-high heat. Add ground beef and cook, stirring to break it up into small pieces, until well browned, about 4 minutes. Add Italian seasoning, garlic powder, onion powder and pepper; cook, stirring, until fragrant, about 30 seconds.

3. Add water, marinara and noodles; bring to a simmer. Cook, covered and stirring often to prevent sticking, until the noodles are tender, about 15 minutes. Stir in Parmesan, basil and parsley.

4. Top with mozzarella (or provolone) and broil until the cheese is bubbly and browned, 2 to 3 minutes. Dollop with ricotta. Garnish with additional basil, if desired.

Prep Time: 20 mins

Total Time: 20 mins

Servings: 4

Ingredients

- 1 pound chicken cutlets
- ½ teaspoon salt, divided
- ½ teaspoon ground pepper, divided
- 1 tablespoon extra-virgin olive oil
- 3 large cloves garlic, grated
- ½ cup dry white wine
- 2 cups coarsely chopped fresh spinach
- ½ cup heavy cream

Directions

1. Sprinkle chicken with 1/4 teaspoon each salt and pepper. Heat oil in a large skillet over medium heat. Add the chicken and cook, turning once, until browned and cooked through, about 6 minutes. Transfer to a plate.

2. Add garlic to the pan and cook, stirring, for 30 seconds. Increase heat to medium-high and add wine. Cook until slightly reduced, about 1 minute. Return heat to medium and stir in spinach, cream and the remaining 1/4 teaspoon each salt and pepper. Simmer for 2 minutes. Return the chicken to the pan and turn to coat with the sauce.b

Prep Time: 30 mins

Total Time: 30 mins

Servings: 4

Ingredients

- 1 pound peeled and deveined jumbo shrimp, thawed if frozen
- 1 teaspoon paprika
- ½ teaspoon garlic powder
- ½ teaspoon dried oregano, crushed
- ¼ teaspoon ground pepper
- ⅛ teaspoon cayenne pepper
- 1 cup whole-grain orzo
- 3 scallions
- 2 tablespoons olive oil, divided
- 2 cups coarsely chopped zucchini
- 1 cup coarsely chopped bell pepper
- ½ cup thinly sliced celery
- 1 cup cherry tomatoes, halved
- ½ teaspoon salt

- 2 tablespoons barbecue sauce
- Lemon wedges for serving

Directions

1. Place shrimp in a medium bowl. Combine paprika, garlic powder, oregano, pepper and cayenne in a small bowl. Sprinkle the spice mixture over the shrimp; toss to coat and set aside.

2. Bring a large saucepan of water to a boil. Cook orzo according to package directions; drain. Return to the hot pot; cover and keep warm.

3. Meanwhile, slice scallions, separating white and green parts. Heat 1 tablespoon oil in a medium skillet over medium-high heat. Add the scallion whites, zucchini, bell pepper and celery; cook, stirring occasionally, until the vegetables are crisp-tender, about 5 minutes. Add tomatoes; cook until softened, 2 to 3 minutes more. Add the vegetables to the pot with the orzo. Add salt; toss to combine.

4. In same skillet, heat the remaining 1 tablespoon oil over medium heat. Add the shrimp; cook, turning once, until opaque, 4 to 6 minutes. Drizzle with

barbecue sauce. Cook and stir until the shrimp are coated, about 1 minute.

5. Serve the shrimp with the vegetable mixture. Top with scallion greens and serve with lemon wedges, if desired.

9. Baked Spinach & Feta Pasta

Prep Time: 10 mins

Total Time: 50 mins

Servings: 4

Ingredients

- 1 (5-ounce) block feta cheese
- 8 cups lightly packed baby spinach (about 5 ounces)
- 3 tablespoons extra-virgin olive oil
- 2 large cloves garlic, minced
- 1 teaspoon dried dill
- ¼ teaspoon kosher salt
- ¼ teaspoon ground pepper
- 8 ounces penne or rotini
- 2 cups boiling water

Directions

1. Preheat oven to 400°F.
2. Place feta in the center of a 9-by-13-inch baking dish. Bake until softened and starting to brown, about 15 minutes.

3. Meanwhile, combine spinach, oil, garlic, dill, salt and pepper in a large bowl. Use your hands to massage the spinach until it's reduced in volume by half. Stir in pasta.

4. After the feta has baked for 15 minutes, add the spinach and pasta mixture to the baking dish. Pour boiling water over the mixture and gently stir. Cover with foil and bake until the pasta is tender, about 18 minutes. Remove from the oven and stir. Cover and let stand for at least 3 minutes before serving.

10. Chicken Parmesan & Quinoa Stuffed Peppers

Prep Time: 15 mins

Total Time: 1 hr

Servings: 4

Ingredients

- 1 tablespoon olive oil
- 1 medium onion, chopped (about 1 1/2 cups)
- 4 cloves garlic, minced
- 1 cup quinoa, rinsed
- 1 ¼ cups water
- 3 cups shredded cooked chicken breast
- 1 ½ cups lower-sodium marinara sauce
- ⅓ cup grated Parmesan cheese
- ¾ cup sliced fresh basil, divided
- 4 large red bell peppers (about 8 ounces each)
- 2 ounces low-moisture, part-skim mozzarella cheese, shredded (about 1/2 cup)

Directions

1. Preheat oven to 350 degrees F. Heat oil in a medium saucepan over medium-high heat. Add

onion and garlic; cook, stirring occasionally, until the onion is translucent, 4 to 5 minutes. Add quinoa; cook, stirring occasionally, for 30 seconds. Add water; increase heat to high and bring to a boil. Reduce heat to medium; cover and cook for 15 minutes. Remove from heat; let stand, covered, for 5 minutes. Stir in chicken, marinara, Parmesan and 1/2 cup basil.

2. Trim top 1/2 inch from peppers; remove seeds and membranes. Arrange the peppers, cut-sides up, in an 8-inch-square glass baking dish. Cover with plastic wrap; microwave on High for 3 minutes. Remove plastic wrap. Spoon the quinoa mixture evenly into the pepper halves (about 1 1/4 cups each).

3. Bake the stuffed peppers until they are softened, about 15 minutes. Sprinkle evenly with mozzarella. Continue baking until the cheese is melted, 5 to 7 minutes. Sprinkle evenly with the remaining 1/4 cup basil.

11. Air-Fryer Lemony Lamb Chops with Fennel & Olives

Prep Time: 15 mins

Total Time: 25 mins

Servings: 2

Ingredients

- 4 teaspoons lemon zest, divided, plus lemon wedges for serving
- ½ teaspoon salt
- ¼ teaspoon ground pepper
- 4 lamb loin chops
- 8 ounces baby yellow potatoes, scrubbed and halved
- 1 fennel bulb, trimmed (2-3 tablespoons fronds reserved and chopped), quartered, cored and sliced
- 1 tablespoon extra-virgin olive oil
- ¼ cup Kalamata olives, chopped

Directions

1. Lightly coat the basket of a 6- to 9-quart air fryer with cooking spray. Preheat to 380°F for 5 minutes.

2. Combine 2 teaspoons lemon zest, salt and pepper in a large bowl. Rub half the mixture over lamb chops. Add potatoes, sliced fennel and oil to the remaining lemon zest mixture in the bowl; toss to coat.

3. Working in batches as necessary, arrange the chops and vegetables in a single layer in the prepared basket.

4. Cook, flipping once, until an instant-read thermometer inserted in the center of a chop registers 145°F, 10 to 12 minutes.

5. Meanwhile, toss olives, the reserved fennel fronds and the remaining 2 teaspoons lemon zest in a bowl. Top the chops and vegetables with the olive mixture. Serve with lemon wedges, if desired.

Prep Time: 30 mins

Total Time: 40 mins

Servings: 6

Ingredients

- 2 tablespoons extra-virgin olive oil
- 1 medium onion, chopped
- 2 cloves garlic, minced
- ⅓ cup tomato paste
- ¼ cup dry white wine
- 1 28-ounce can no-salt-added whole peeled tomatoes, preferably San Marzano
- 3 cups cooked corona beans or two 15-ounce cans no-salt-added cannellini beans, rinsed
- 2 tablespoons chopped fresh basil, plus more for garnish
- 2 tablespoons chopped fresh oregano, plus more for garnish
- 2 tablespoons chopped fresh parsley, plus more for garnish
- 1 large egg, lightly beaten

- ⅔ cup whole-milk ricotta cheese

- ½ cup grated Parmesan cheese, divided

- 1 cup shredded fontina cheese

Directions

1. Heat oil in a large oven-safe skillet over medium-high heat. Add onion and cook, stirring occasionally, until softened, about 5 minutes. Add garlic and cook, stirring, until fragrant, about 1 minute. Add tomato paste and cook, stirring, until it starts to darken, about 2 minutes. Add wine and cook, scraping up any browned bits, until thickened, about 1 minute. Add tomatoes and their juice, crushing the tomatoes with your hand as you add them. Stir in beans, basil, oregano and parsley. Bring to a simmer. Reduce heat to maintain a simmer and cook, stirring occasionally, until thickened, 18 to 20 minutes.

2. Meanwhile, place rack in upper third of oven; preheat broiler to high. Combine egg, ricotta and 1/4 cup Parmesan in a small bowl.

3. Gently stir the ricotta mixture into the bean mixture. Sprinkle fontina and the remaining 1/4

cup Parmesan on top. Broil until the cheese is melted, 2 to 3 minutes. Garnish with more herbs, if desired.

Prep Time: 45 mins

Total Time: 45 mins

Servings: 4

Ingredients

- 3 cups water
- ¾ cup whole milk
- ¾ cup grits or polenta
- ⅓ cup grated Parmesan cheese
- ¾ teaspoon kosher salt, divided
- ½ teaspoon ground pepper, divided
- 2 tablespoons extra-virgin olive oil, divided
- 1 large onion, chopped
- 3 cloves garlic, sliced
- 1 (14 ounce) can no-salt-added fire-roasted diced tomatoes
- 3 teaspoons smoked paprika, divided
- 2 pounds collards, stemmed and thinly sliced
- 1 pound raw shrimp (31-35 count), peeled and deveined

Directions

1. Combine water and milk in a large saucepan; bring to a boil. Whisk in grits (or polenta) until smooth. Cover and reduce heat to low. Cook, whisking occasionally, until creamy and thickened, about 25 minutes. Remove from heat.

2. Stir in Parmesan, 1/2 teaspoon salt and 1/4 teaspoon pepper. Cover and set aside.

3. Meanwhile, heat 1 tablespoon oil in a large high-sided skillet or large pot over medium heat. Add onion and cook, stirring occasionally, until soft, about 3 minutes. Add garlic and cook for 1 minute. Stir in tomatoes, 2 teaspoons paprika and the remaining 1/4 teaspoon each salt and pepper. Add collards by the handful, letting them wilt slightly after each addition. Continue to cook, stirring frequently, until the collards are tender and beginning to darken, about 10 minutes. Transfer to a bowl and cover to keep warm.

4. Add the remaining 1 tablespoon oil to the pan and increase heat to medium-high. Toss shrimp with the remaining 1 teaspoon paprika in a medium

bowl. Add the shrimp to the pan and cook, stirring occasionally, until they turn pink, 3 to 4 minutes.

5. Serve the shrimp and collards with the grits.

14. Crispy Rice Bowls with Fried Eggs

Prep Time: 25 mins

Total Time: 25 mins

Servings: 4

Ingredients

- 2 teaspoons toasted sesame oil, divided
- 2 ½ cups cooked brown rice
- ½ teaspoon salt plus a pinch, divided
- 2 tablespoons grapeseed or canola oil, divided
- 1 teaspoon grated fresh ginger
- 1 11-ounce package baby spinach
- 1 tablespoon lime juice
- 4 large eggs
- 1 ripe avocado, sliced
- 1 cup julienned carrot
- 4 radishes, thinly sliced
- 2 scallions, thinly sliced
- 4 teaspoons Sriracha

Directions

1. Heat 1 teaspoon sesame oil in a large nonstick skillet over medium-high heat. Add rice and sprinkle with 1/4 teaspoon salt; cook, stirring occasionally, until crispy, about 10 minutes. Divide among 4 shallow bowls.

2. Add the remaining 1 teaspoon sesame oil, 1 tablespoon grapeseed (or canola) oil and ginger to the pan. Add spinach, in batches, and cook, tossing, until wilted, 2 to 3 minutes. Stir in lime juice and 1/4 teaspoon salt. Divide among the rice bowls.

3. Heat the remaining 1 tablespoon grapeseed (or canola) oil in the pan. Crack eggs into it and cook until the whites are set and the edges are crispy, about 3 minutes. Sprinkle with the remaining pinch of salt. Place an egg on each rice bowl. Top with avocado, carrot, radishes, scallions and Sriracha.

15. 25-Minute Chicken & Veggie Enchiladas

Prep Time: 25 mins

Total Time: 25 mins

Servings: 4

Ingredients

- 2 tablespoons canola oil
- 1 ½ cups chopped zucchini
- 1 ½ cups chopped yellow squash
- ½ cup chopped yellow onion
- 1 teaspoon minced garlic
- 1 ½ cups shredded, cooked chicken breast (about 4 1/2 oz.)
- ½ cup shredded, cooked chicken thigh (about 1 1/2 oz.)
- ⅝ teaspoon kosher salt
- ½ teaspoon black pepper
- 4 ounces Monterey Jack cheese, shredded (about 1 cup), divided
- 8 (6 inch) corn tortillas
- Cooking spray
- ½ cup bottled salsa verde

- Fresh cilantro leaves

Directions

1. Preheat oven to broil with rack 5 to 6 inches from heat. Heat oil in a large nonstick skillet over medium-high. Add zucchini, squash, and onion, and cook, stirring often, until vegetables are tender and just beginning to brown, about 10 minutes. Add garlic, and cook 1 more minute. Add chicken, salt, pepper, and 3/4 cup of the cheese; stir to combine. Cook until hot and cheese melts, about 1 minute. Remove from heat, and cover to keep warm.

2. Warm tortillas according to package directions. Place about 1/3 cup of chicken mixture in center of each tortilla; fold tortilla around filling, and place, seam side down, in a lightly greased (with cooking spray) 11- x 7-inch (or a 2-quart) broiler-safe baking dish. Pour salsa over enchiladas, and sprinkle with remaining 1/4 cup cheese. Broil in preheated oven until hot and bubbly, about 1 1/2 minutes. Garnish with cilantro.

Prep Time: 1 hr

Total Time: 4 hrs

Servings: 12

Ingredients

- 2 tablespoons extra-virgin olive oil, plus more for serving
- 2 tablespoons unsalted butter
- 2 leeks, white and light green parts only, rinsed and diced
- 2 cloves garlic, roughly chopped
- 2 teaspoons salt, divided
- Ground pepper to taste
- 1 pound potatoes, diced (1/2-inch)
- 3 medium carrots, sliced 1/4-inch thick
- 4 celery stalks, sliced 1/4-inch thick
- 2 medium yellow squash, halved lengthwise and sliced 1/4-inch thick
- 1 medium zucchini, halved lengthwise and sliced 1/4-inch thick

- 8 ounces green beans, trimmed and cut into 1/2-inch pieces
- 1 pound frozen or fresh (shelled) peas
- 3 ½ cups cooked beans with their cooking liquid clinging to them, such as cannellini and/or kidney beans or 2 (15- ounce) cans beans, drained but not rinsed
- 4 cups water or 2 cups water and 2 cups homemade chicken stock
- 1 (2 inch) piece Parmesan rind
- 1 (28 ounce) can whole peeled tomatoes with juice
- 1 pound pasta, such as orecchiette or medium shells
- Roughly torn fresh basil and grated Parmigiano-Reggiano for serving

Directions

1. Heat oil and butter in a large pot over medium-low heat (the goal is to build flavor slowly at first). When the butter has melted, add leeks and garlic and season with a pinch each of salt and pepper. Cook, stirring occasionally (and get used to this

step, since you are going to be doing it every time you add a new ingredient) until they have wilted and softened, about 4 minutes.

2. Remark over how wonderful the kitchen smells, then add potatoes and a pinch each of salt and pepper. Stir to combine, and cook until the potatoes begin to sizzle. Add carrots and a pinch each of salt and pepper and stir. By now the pan will start to be crowded, so you can increase the heat to medium.

3. Repeat these steps while adding each new ingredient, seasoning, stirring and allowing to sizzle before moving on to the next, adding in this order: celery, yellow squash, zucchini, green beans and peas. It should almost look like you are making a vegetable potpie filling.

4. Add beans and the liquid clinging to them. Add a pinch each of salt and pepper. Add water (or water and stock). Increase heat to medium-high and add Parmesan rind. Cook, stirring occasionally, until the soup comes to a simmer. Add tomatoes and their juices and a pinch each of salt and pepper; bring to a gentle simmer.

5. Reduce heat to a bare simmer and cover the pot. Continue simmering, stirring occasionally, until it has thickened into a hearty stew, about 3 hours. Taste for seasoning and adjust as you see fit.

6. Just before serving, cook pasta according to package directions. Drain.

7. Serve the soup with the pasta. Top with cheese and basil and a drizzle of olive oil, if desired.

Prep Time: 35 mins

Total Time: 35 mins

Servings: 4

Ingredients

- 4 cloves garlic, finely chopped
- ¾ teaspoon salt, divided
- ¼ cup lemon juice
- 1 teaspoon ground cumin
- 1 teaspoon paprika
- ½ teaspoon ground pepper
- 1 pound boneless, skinless chicken breasts, trimmed, cut into 1-inch pieces
- 1 tablespoon extra-virgin olive oil
- 1 large yellow onion, chopped
- 1 14-ounce can no-salt-added diced tomatoes
- 1 15-ounce can chickpeas, rinsed
- ¼ cup chopped flat-leaf parsley

Directions

1. Mash garlic and 1/2 teaspoon salt on a cutting board with the back of a fork until a paste forms. Transfer to a medium bowl and whisk in lemon juice, cumin, paprika and pepper. Add chicken and stir to coat.

2. Heat oil in a large cast-iron skillet over medium-high heat. Add onion and cook, stirring occasionally, until golden brown, 6 to 8 minutes. Using a slotted spoon, transfer the chicken to the pan (reserve the marinade) and cook, stirring occasionally, until opaque on the outside, about 4 minutes. Add tomatoes with their juice, chickpeas, the reserved marinade and the remaining 1/4 teaspoon salt. Reduce heat to medium and cook, stirring occasionally, until the chicken is cooked through, 5 to 7 minutes more. Serve sprinkled with parsley.

Prep Time: 30 mins

Total Time: 45 mins

Servings: 4

Ingredients

- 3 teaspoons extra-virgin olive oil, divided
- 1 small onion, finely chopped
- 1 stalk celery, finely diced
- 2 tablespoons chopped fresh parsley
- 15 ounces canned salmon, drained, or 1 1/2 cups cooked salmon
- 1 large egg, lightly beaten
- 1 ½ teaspoons Dijon mustard
- 1 3/4 cups fresh whole-wheat breadcrumbs
- ½ teaspoon freshly ground pepper
- Creamy Dill Sauce
- 1 lemon, cut into wedges

Directions

1. Preheat oven to 450 degrees F. Coat a baking sheet with cooking spray.

2. Heat 1 1/2 teaspoons oil in a large nonstick skillet over medium-high heat. Add onion and celery; cook, stirring, until softened, about 3 minutes. Stir in parsley; remove from the heat.

3. Place salmon in a medium bowl. Flake apart with a fork; remove any bones and skin. Add egg and mustard; mix well. Add the onion mixture, breadcrumbs and pepper; mix well. Shape the mixture into 8 patties, about 2 1/2 inches wide.

4. Heat remaining 1 1/2 teaspoons oil in the pan over medium heat. Add 4 patties and cook until the undersides are golden, 2 to 3 minutes. Using a wide spatula, turn them over onto the prepared baking sheet. Repeat with the remaining patties.

5. Bake the salmon cakes until golden on top and heated through, 15 to 20 minutes. Meanwhile, prepare Creamy Dill Sauce. Serve salmon cakes with sauce and lemon wedges.

19. Butternut Squash & Black Bean Enchiladas

Prep Time: 25 mins

Total Time: 45 mins

Servings: 4

Ingredients

- 3 tablespoons extra-virgin olive oil, divided
- 3 cups diced peeled butternut squash
- 2 medium poblano peppers, seeded and chopped
- 1 medium onion, chopped
- 1 (14 ounce) can no-salt-added black beans, rinsed
- 4 tablespoons chopped fresh cilantro, divided, plus more for serving
- 1 tablespoon ancho chile powder
- 8 corn tortillas, warmed
- 1 (10-ounce) can enchilada sauce
- ½ cup shredded Monterey Jack cheese
- 2 cups shredded cabbage
- 1 tablespoon lime juice

Directions

1. Preheat oven to 425°F. Lightly coat a 7-by-11-inch baking dish with cooking spray.

2. Heat 2 tablespoons oil in a large skillet over medium heat. Add squash and cook, covered, stirring occasionally, until tender and lightly browned, 8 to 10 minutes. Add peppers and onion and cook, uncovered, stirring occasionally, until tender, about 5 minutes. Remove from heat and stir in beans, 2 tablespoons cilantro and chile powder. Let cool for 5 minutes.

3. Place about 1/2 cup of the squash mixture in each tortilla and roll. Place, seam-side down, in the prepared baking dish. Top with enchilada sauce. Sprinkle with cheese and cover with foil. Bake until bubbly, about 15 minutes. Remove foil and bake for another 5 minutes.

4. Meanwhile, toss cabbage with lime juice, the remaining 1 tablespoon oil and 2 tablespoons cilantro. Serve the enchiladas topped with the slaw and more cilantro, if desired.

Prep Time: 25 mins

Total Time: 25 mins

Servings: 4

Ingredients

- 12 ounces beef flank steak, trimmed
- 1 tablespoon minced fresh ginger
- 1 ½ teaspoons reduced-sodium soy sauce
- 1 teaspoon dry sherry plus 1 Tbsp., divided
- 1 teaspoon cornstarch
- 1 teaspoon toasted sesame oil
- 2 tablespoons oyster-flavored sauce, preferably Lee Kum Kee Premium
- 1 tablespoon vegetable oil
- 1 pound baby bok choy, trimmed and cut into 2-inch pieces (about 8 cups)
- 3 tablespoons unsalted chicken broth

Directions

1. Cut beef with the grain into 2-inch-wide strips. Cut each strip across the grain into 1/4-inch-thick

slices. Combine the beef, ginger, soy sauce, 1 tsp. sherry, and cornstarch in a medium bowl; stir until the cornstarch is no longer visible. Add sesame oil and stir until the beef is lightly coated.

2. Combine oyster-flavored sauce and the remaining 1 Tbsp. sherry in a small bowl. Set aside.

3. Heat a 14-inch flat-bottomed carbon-steel wok (or a 12-inch stainless-steel skillet) over high heat until a drop of water vaporizes within 1 to 2 seconds of contact. Swirl in vegetable oil. Add the beef in an even layer; cook, undisturbed, until it begins to brown, about 1 minute. Using a metal spatula, stir-fry until lightly browned but not cooked through, 30 seconds to 1 minute more. Transfer to a plate.

4. Add bok choy and broth to the pan. Cover and cook until the bok choy greens are bright green and almost all the liquid has been absorbed, 1 to 2 minutes. Return the beef to the pan, add the reserved sauce, and stir-fry until the beef is just cooked through and the bok choy is tender-crisp, 30 seconds to 1 minute.

21. Black Bean-Cauliflower Rice Bowl

Prep Time: 20 mins

Total Time: 20 mins

Servings: 1

Ingredients

- 1 tablespoon olive oil plus 2 tsp., divided
- 1 cup frozen cauliflower rice
- ⅛ teaspoon salt
- 2 tablespoons chopped onion
- 2 tablespoons chopped green bell pepper
- ½ teaspoon chili powder
- ½ teaspoon ground cumin
- ¼ teaspoon dried oregano
- ⅔ cup no-salt-added canned black beans, rinsed
- 2 tablespoons chopped roasted red pepper
- ¼ cup water
- 1 tablespoon lime juice
- ¼ cup shredded reduced-fat Cheddar cheese
- 1 medium tomato, chopped
- 1 tablespoon chopped fresh cilantro for garnish

Directions

1. Heat 1 Tbsp. oil in a medium skillet over medium heat. Add cauliflower rice and salt; cook, stirring often, until heated through, 3 to 5 minutes. Transfer to a small bowl and keep warm. Wipe out the pan.

2. Heat the remaining 2 tsp. oil in the pan over medium heat. Add onion, green pepper, chili powder, cumin, and oregano; cook, stirring often, until the vegetables are softened, about 3 minutes. Add beans, roasted red pepper, and water; bring to a simmer. Cook, stirring occasionally, until heated through and thickened, 3 to 5 minutes. Remove from heat. Stir in lime juice.

3. Arrange the bean mixture with the hot cauliflower rice in a dinner bowl. Top with cheese and tomato. Garnish with cilantro, if desired.

Total Time: 30 mins

Servings: 4

Ingredients

- 1 ½ teaspoons dried thyme
- 1 ½ teaspoons ground cumin
- ¼ teaspoon salt
- ¼ teaspoon pepper
- 4 large boneless, skinless chicken thighs (about 1 1/4 pounds), trimmed
- 2 tablespoons extra-virgin olive oil, divided
- 1 medium onion, halved and sliced
- 1 cup Israeli couscous
- 2 cloves garlic, minced
- 4 cups very thinly sliced kale
- 2 cups reduced-sodium chicken broth

Directions

1. Combine thyme, cumin, salt and pepper in a small bowl. Sprinkle both sides of chicken with half of the spice mixture.

2. Heat 1 tablespoon oil in a large, heavy skillet, such as cast-iron, over medium-high heat. Add chicken and cook until golden brown, 2 to 3 minutes per side. Transfer to a plate.

3. Add the remaining 1 tablespoon oil and onion to the pan; cook, stirring frequently, until beginning to soften, 2 to 4 minutes. Stir in couscous and garlic; cook, stirring frequently, until the couscous is lightly toasted, 1 to 2 minutes. Add kale and the remaining spice mixture; cook, stirring, until the kale begins to wilt, 1 to 2 minutes.

4. Pour in broth and any accumulated juice from the chicken, then nestle the chicken into the couscous. Reduce the heat to medium-low, cover and cook until the chicken is cooked through and the couscous is tender, 10 to 12 minutes.

23. Garlic Green Beans with Crispy Ground Beef

Prep Time: 25 mins

Total Time: 25 mins

Servings: 4

Ingredients

- 3 tablespoons canola oil, divided
- 8 ounces 90%-lean ground beef
- ½ teaspoon salt, divided
- 2 tablespoons rice vinegar
- 2 tablespoons Shaoxing rice wine or dry sherry
- 1 tablespoon toasted sesame oil
- 1 ½ teaspoons fish sauce
- 1 teaspoon granulated sugar
- ½ teaspoon ground white pepper
- 1 ½ pounds green beans, trimmed and halved
- ½ cup sliced scallion whites, plus sliced scallion greens for garnish
- 6 cloves garlic, minced
- 2 teaspoons grated fresh ginger

Directions

1. Heat 1 tablespoon canola oil in a large flat-bottom
    wok or skillet over medium-high heat. Add beef
    and cook, breaking into large pieces with a wooden
    spoon, until well browned and crispy, 4 to 6
    minutes. Sprinkle with 1/4 teaspoon salt, then
    transfer to a small bowl.

2. Meanwhile, whisk vinegar, Shaoxing (or sherry),
    sesame oil, fish sauce, sugar and white pepper in a
    small bowl. Set next to the stove.

3. Heat the remaining 2 tablespoons canola oil in the
    pan. Add green beans and cook, stirring
    occasionally, until slightly charred and tender, 4 to
    6 minutes. Add scallion whites, garlic and ginger;
    cook, stirring, until fragrant, about 1 minute. Add
    the vinegar mixture, reserved beef and remaining
    1/4 teaspoon salt; cook, stirring, until well coated,
    about 1 minute. Serve sprinkled with scallion
    greens, if desired.

24. Chicken Cutlets with Roasted Red Pepper & Arugula Relish

Prep Time: 20 mins

Total Time: 20 mins

Servings: 4

Ingredients

- 1 pound chicken cutlets
- ¾ teaspoon sweet or hot Hungarian paprika
- ½ teaspoon ground pepper, divided
- ⅛ teaspoon salt plus a pinch, divided
- 1 tablespoon extra-virgin olive oil
- 1 tablespoon dried currants
- 2 tablespoons warm water
- ½ cup chopped arugula
- ½ cup jarred roasted red peppers, rinsed and finely chopped
- 1 tablespoon pine nuts, toasted
- 1 ½ teaspoons granulated sugar
- ½ clove garlic, grated
- 1 teaspoon sherry vinegar

Directions

1. Sprinkle chicken with paprika, 1/4 teaspoon pepper and 1/8 teaspoon salt. Heat oil in a large skillet over medium-high heat until shimmering. Add the chicken and cook, flipping halfway, until golden brown and an instant-read thermometer inserted in the thickest part registers 165°F, 6 to 8 minutes. Transfer to a plate.

2. Meanwhile, soak currants in water for 5 minutes; drain. Combine the currants, arugula, roasted peppers, pine nuts, sugar, garlic, vinegar and the remaining 1/4 teaspoon pepper and pinch of salt in a small bowl. Serve with the chicken.

Total Time: 20 mins

Servings: 4

Ingredients

- 8 ounces whole-wheat spaghetti
- 3 tablespoons toasted (dark) sesame oil
- 2 scallions, chopped
- 1 tablespoon minced garlic
- 2 teaspoons minced fresh ginger
- 1 teaspoon brown sugar
- 2 tablespoons reduced-sodium soy sauce
- 2 tablespoons ketchup
- 8 ounces cooked boneless, skinless chicken breast, shredded
- 1 cup julienned carrots
- 1 cup sliced snap peas
- 3 tablespoons toasted sesame seeds

Directions

1. Cook spaghetti in a pot of boiling water according to package directions. Drain, rinse and transfer to a large bowl.

2. Combine sesame oil, scallions, garlic, ginger and brown sugar in a small saucepan. Heat over medium heat until starting to sizzle. Cook for 15 seconds. Remove from heat and stir in soy sauce and ketchup. Add to the noodles along with chicken, carrots, snap peas and sesame seeds; gently toss to combine.

26. Philly Cheesesteak Stuffed Peppers

Prep Time: 40 mins

Total Time: 40 mins

Servings: 4

Ingredients

- 2 large bell peppers, halved lengthwise, seeds removed
- 1 tablespoon extra-virgin olive oil
- 1 large onion, halved and sliced
- 1 (8 ounce) package mushrooms, thinly sliced
- 12 ounces top round steak, thinly sliced
- 1 tablespoon Italian seasoning
- ½ teaspoon ground pepper
- ¼ teaspoon salt
- 1 tablespoon Worcestershire sauce
- 4 slices provolone cheese

Directions

1. Preheat oven to 375 degrees F.

2. Place pepper halves on a rimmed baking sheet. Bake until tender but still holding their shape, about 30 minutes.

3. Meanwhile, heat oil in a large skillet over medium heat. Add onion and cook, stirring, until starting to brown, 4 to 5 minutes. Add mushrooms and cook, stirring, until they're softened and release their juices, about 5 minutes more. Add steak, Italian seasoning, pepper and salt; cook, stirring, until the steak is just cooked through, 3 to 5 minutes more. Remove from heat and stir in Worcestershire.

4. Preheat broiler to high. Divide the filling between the pepper halves and top each with a slice of cheese. Broil 5 inches from the heat until the cheese is melted and lightly browned, 2 to 3 minutes.

27. Black Bean-Quinoa Bowl

Prep Time: 10 mins

Total Time: 10 mins

Servings: 1

Ingredients

- ¾ cup canned black beans, rinsed
- ⅔ cup cooked quinoa
- ¼ cup hummus
- 1 tablespoon lime juice
- ¼ medium avocado, diced
- 3 tablespoons pico de gallo
- 2 tablespoons chopped fresh cilantro

Directions

1. Combine beans and quinoa in a bowl. Stir hummus and lime juice together in a small bowl; thin with water to desired consistency. Drizzle the hummus dressing over the beans and quinoa. Top with avocado, pico de gallo and cilantro.

28. Creamy Spinach Pasta

Prep Time: 15 mins

Total Time: 15 mins

Servings: 4

Ingredients

- 12 ounces uncooked tube-shaped chickpea pasta (about 3 1/2 cups) (such as Banza)
- 1 clove garlic, thinly sliced (about 1 tsp.)
- 2 tablespoons thinly sliced shallots
- 3 ¼ ounces mascarpone cheese
- 4 ounces fresh baby spinach
- 1 teaspoon kosher salt
- ½ teaspoon black pepper
- 1 teaspoon lemon zest (from 1 lemon)
- 1 pinch Crushed red pepper

Directions

1. Cook pasta according to package directions, omitting salt. Drain, reserving 1 cup cooking water.
2. Transfer pasta to a large bowl; add garlic, shallot, mascarpone, spinach, salt, pepper, and 1/2 cup of

the reserved cooking liquid. Stir until cheese has melted and mixture is combined, about 1 1/2 minutes. Add additional cooking liquid as needed to loosen sauce. Divide pasta among 4 bowls. Sprinkle with lemon zest and, if desired, crushed red pepper. Serve immediately.

Prep Time: 15 mins

Total Time: 1 hr 30 mins

Servings: 8

Ingredients

- 2 tablespoons extra-virgin olive oil
- ¾ cup finely chopped yellow onion
- ½ cup finely chopped celery
- 1 tablespoon finely chopped garlic
- 1 ½ pounds 90%-lean ground beef
- ½ pound mild Italian turkey sausage
- 1 cup whole-wheat panko breadcrumbs
- ¾ cup lower-sodium ketchup, divided
- ¼ cup chopped fresh flat-leaf parsley plus 1 tablespoon, divided
- ¼ cup grated Parmesan cheese
- 2 large egg, lightly beaten
- 1 ½ tablespoons dried Italian seasoning
- ¾ teaspoon salt
- ½ teaspoon ground pepper

Directions

1. Position oven rack about 8 inches from broiler; preheat to 350°F. Lightly coat a 9-by-5-inch loaf pan with cooking spray.

2. Heat oil in a medium skillet over medium-high heat. Add onion, celery and garlic; cook, stirring often, until the vegetables are slightly softened, about 4 minutes. Remove from heat and allow to cool slightly.

3. Transfer the cooled onion mixture to a large bowl. Add beef, sausage, panko, 1/2 cup ketchup, 1/4 cup parsley, Parmesan, eggs, Italian seasoning, salt and pepper; gently but thoroughly mix with your hands until well combined. Transfer to the prepared pan, packing the mixture tightly so no air pockets exist. Spoon the remaining 1/4 cup ketchup over the top, spreading in an even layer.

4. Bake until a thermometer inserted in the thickest portion registers 165°F, about 1 hour. Increase oven temperature to broil; broil until the top is lightly browned, 6 to 8 minutes. Let stand at room temperature for 10 minutes before using a spatula

to lift the meatloaf out of the pan, allowing any liquid to drain away. Place on a platter or work surface; slice into 8 portions. Sprinkle with the remaining 1 tablespoon parsley.

Prep Time: 5 mins

Total Time: 5 mins

Servings: 6

Ingredients

- 1 large cucumber, unpeeled, halved and seeded
- ¾ cup whole-milk plain yogurt
- 2 teaspoons chopped fresh dill
- 1 small clove garlic, grated
- ½ teaspoon grated lemon zest
- ½ teaspoon salt
- Freshly ground black pepper to taste

Directions

1. Coarsely shred cucumber over a clean kitchen towel. Wrap the towel around the shredded cucumber; gently squeeze to remove excess liquid. Transfer the cucumber to a medium bowl.
2. Add yogurt, dill, garlic, lemon zest and salt; stir to combine. Season with pepper to taste.